Copyright Page

Copyright 2020 Andre Calbert

All rights reserved. No part of this publication may be reproduced, distributed, or transmitted in any form or by any means, including photocopying, recording, or other electronic or mechanical methods, without the prior written permission of the publisher, except in the case of brief quotations embodied in critical reviews and certain other noncommercial uses permitted by copyright law. For permission requests, please contact the publisher or author.

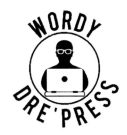

Disclaimer

This is a work of fiction. Any resemblance to actual events or persons, living or dead, is entirely coincidental.

ISBN 978-1-7351715-1-7

Version- Printed Soft Cover

This book is dedicated to all the moms and dads out there who are fighting every day to teach their kids about the importance of brushing their teeth, eating healthy, and maintaining good oral hygiene. As a single parent myself, I also struggled with these very issues when raising my child. You may teach them one thing, and then they may experience a different set of rules while visiting another household. It could be the other parent, or an aunt, or grandma's house or another relative or friend. The goal of this book is for these healthy habits to become ingrained so that the child carries them wherever they may go.

Tooth Fairy Wishes

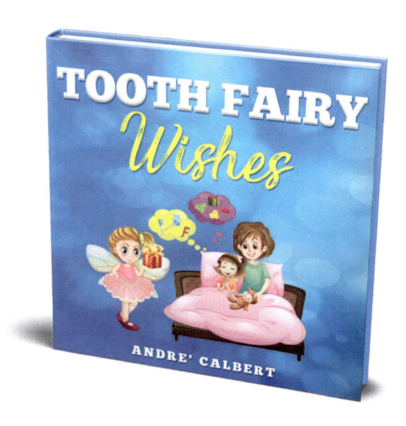

by Andre' Calbert

Illustrations by Aneeza Ashraf

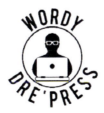

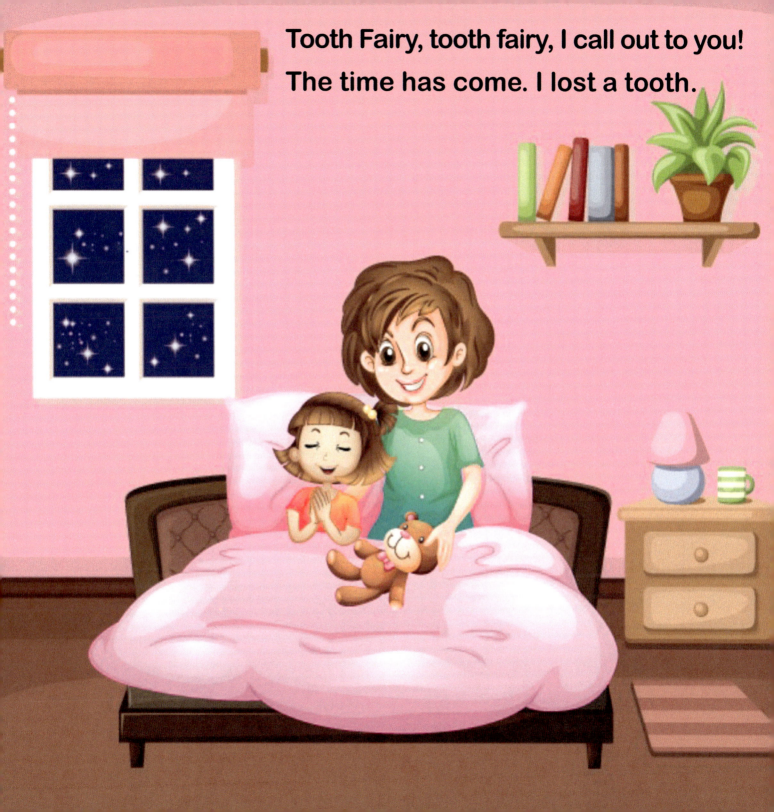

Tooth Fairy, tooth fairy, I call out to you!
The time has come. I lost a tooth.

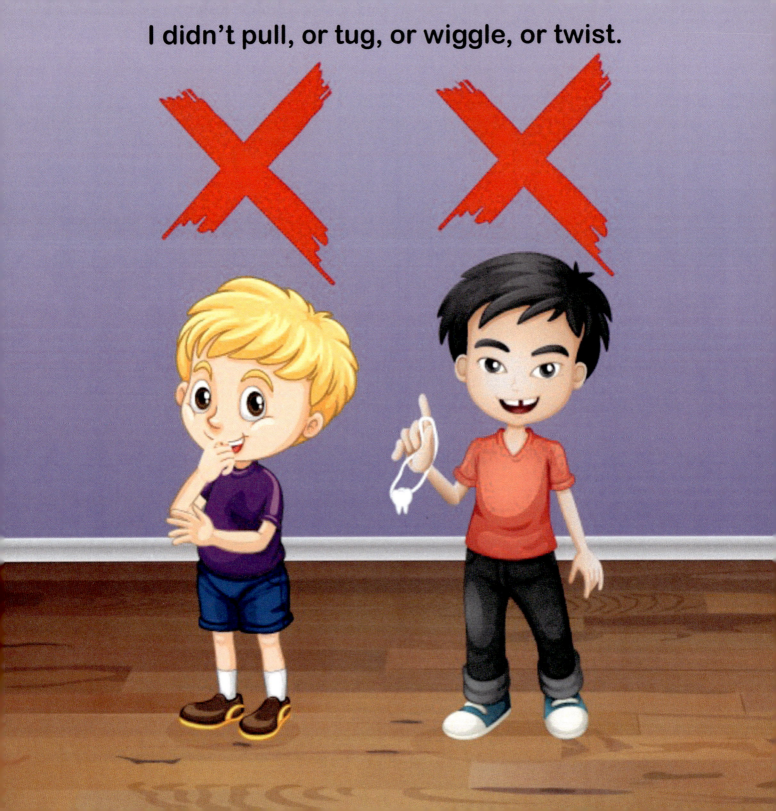

My tooth came loose on its own. I insist!

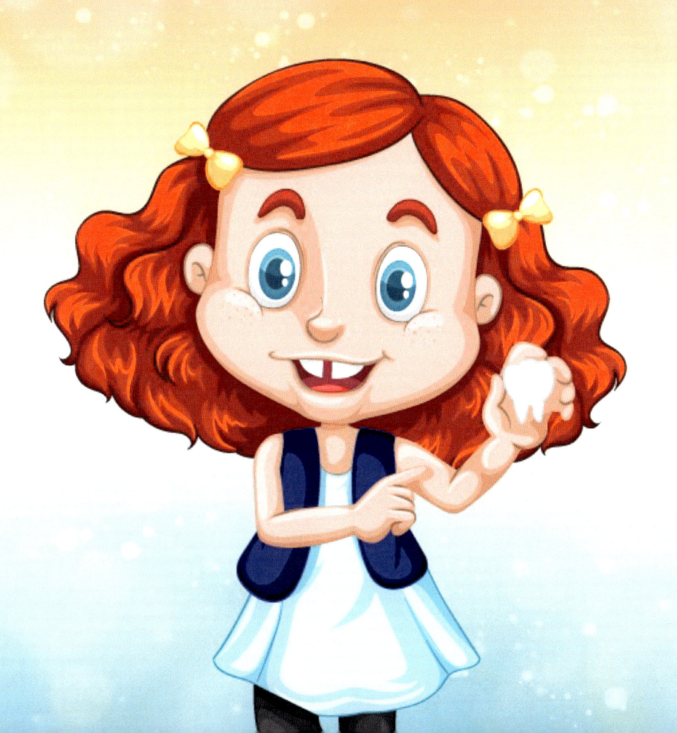

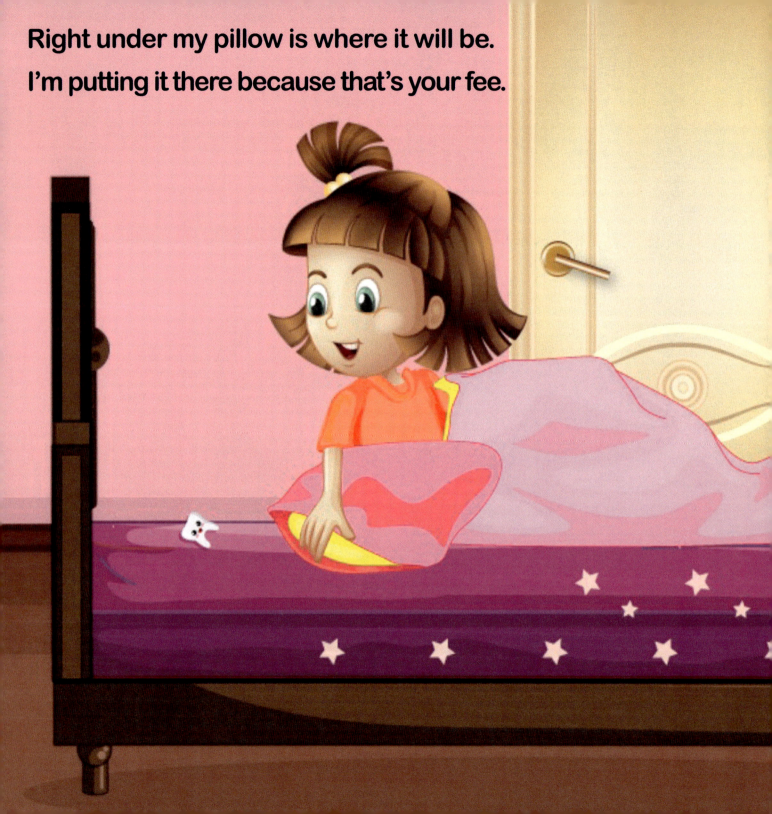
Right under my pillow is where it will be.
I'm putting it there because that's your fee.

I'll trade and exchange my tooth for a gift.
I won't get to see you cause you're fast and you're swift.

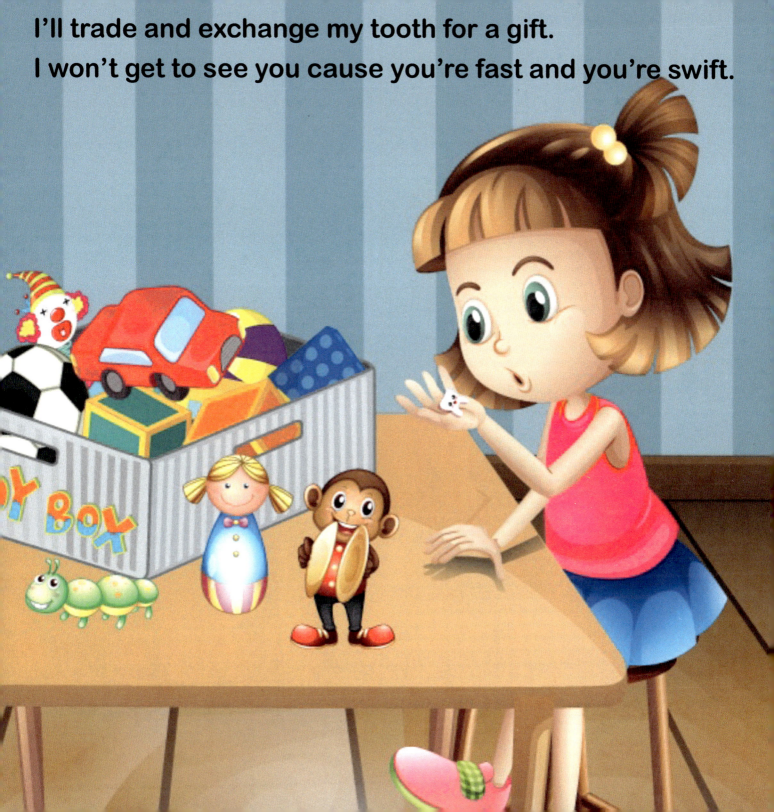

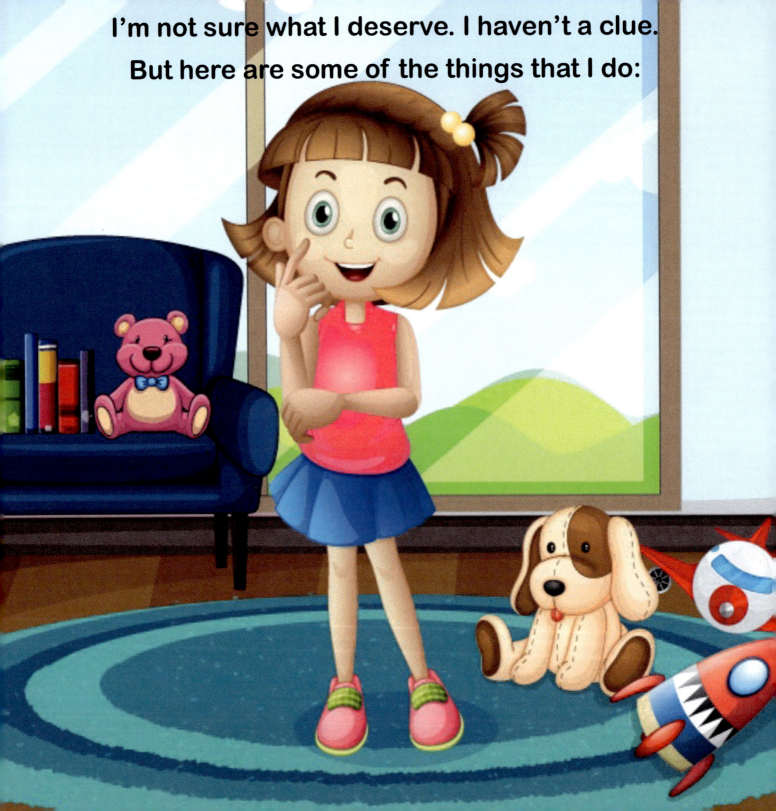

I'm not sure what I deserve. I haven't a clue.
But here are some of the things that I do:

Each night before bed, I brush really good just like my parents say that I should.
And when I wake up, I do the same.
I brush and brush and brush again.

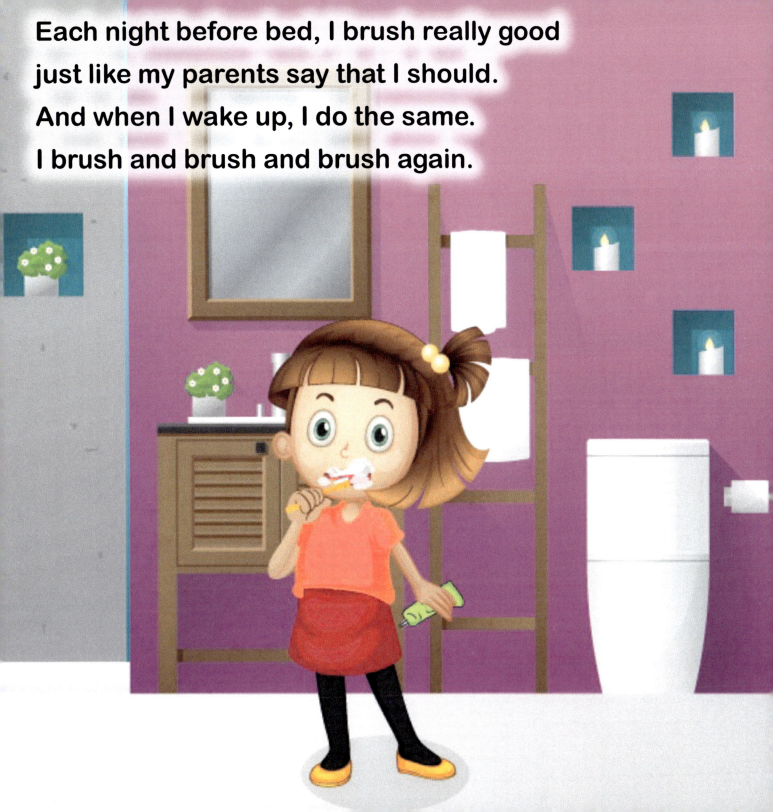

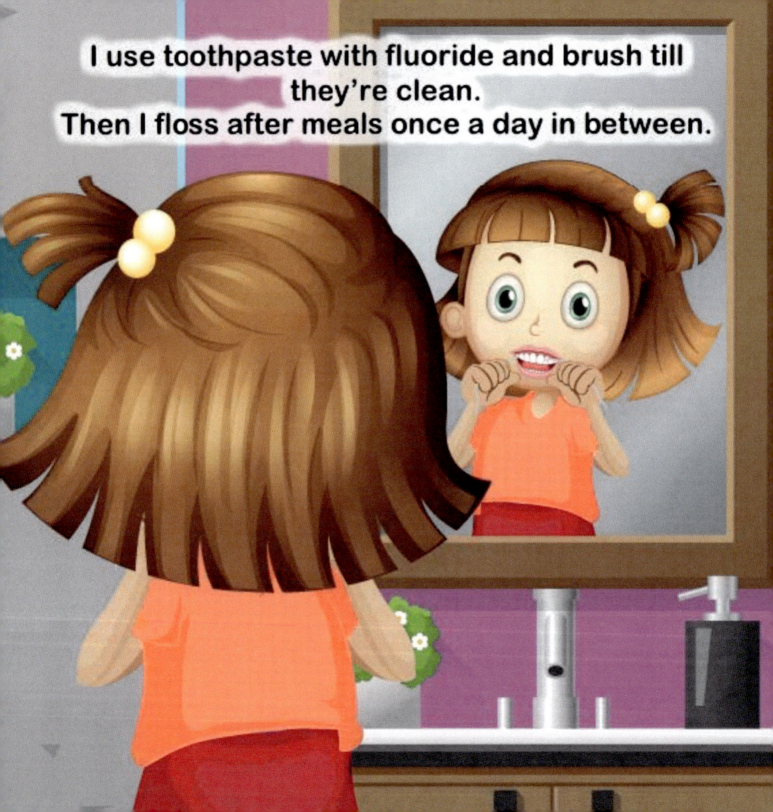

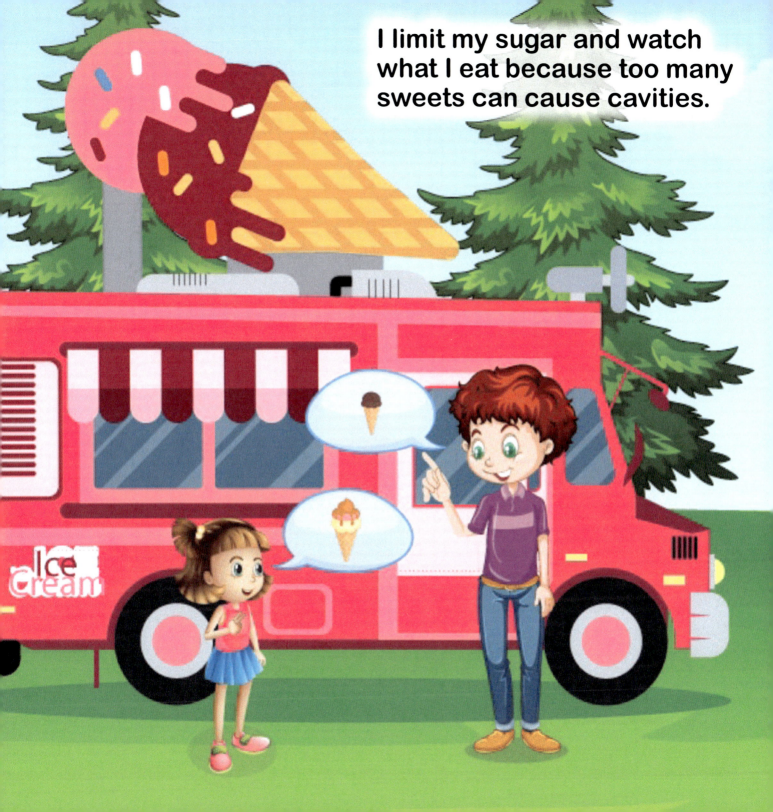

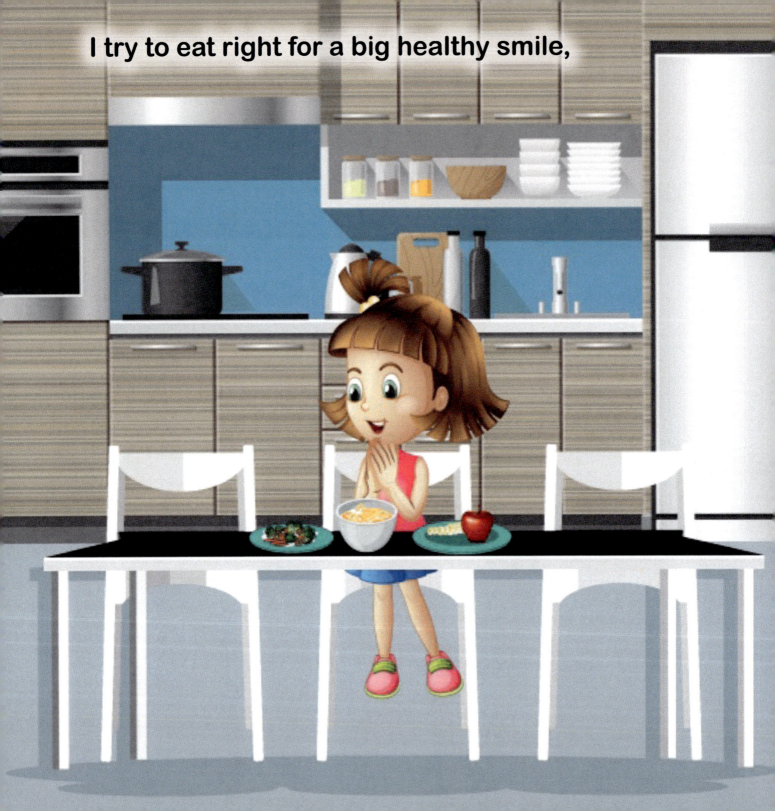

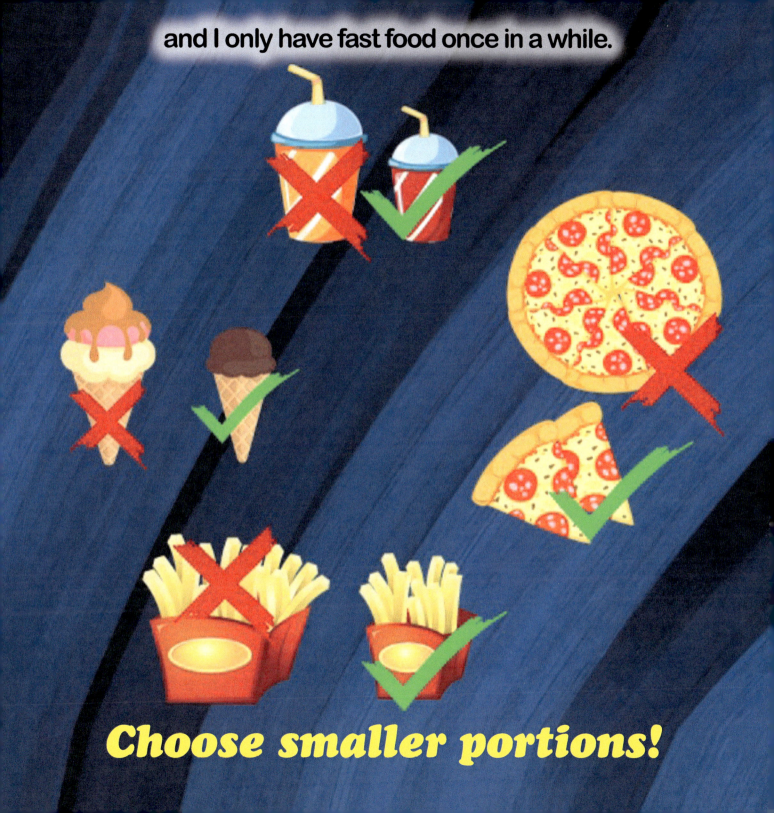

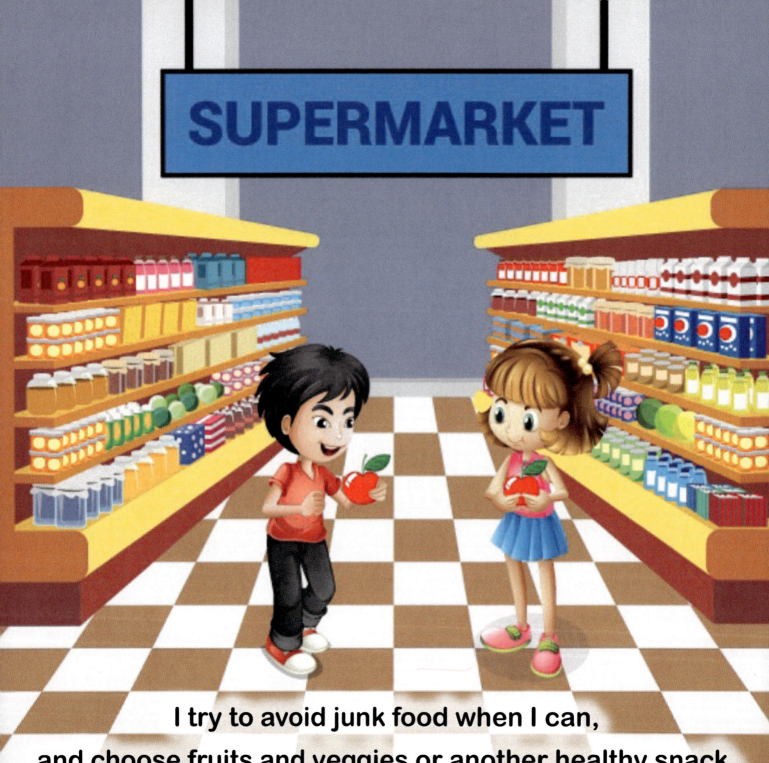

I try to avoid junk food when I can,
and choose fruits and veggies or another healthy snack.

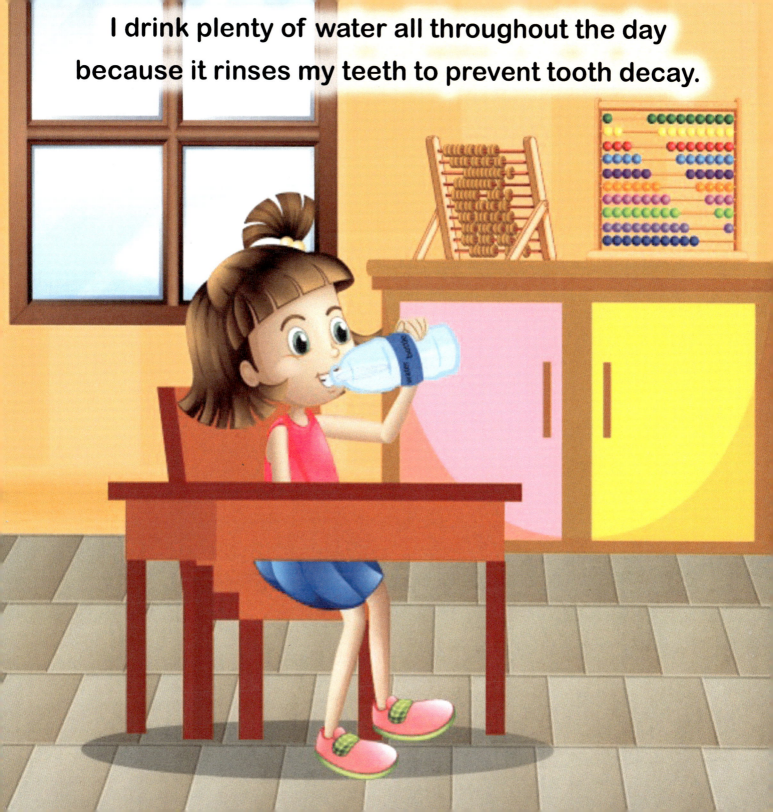

I drink plenty of water all throughout the day because it rinses my teeth to prevent tooth decay.

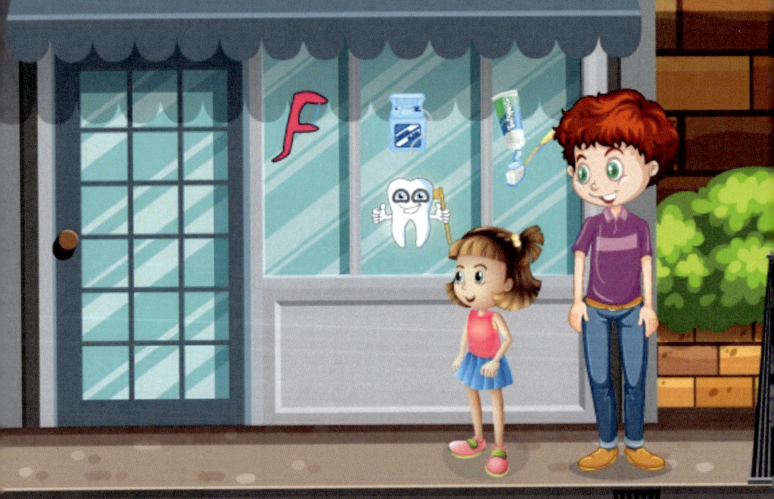

I get regular check-ups to see how I've done.
I say "aah", and the dentist looks under my tongue.

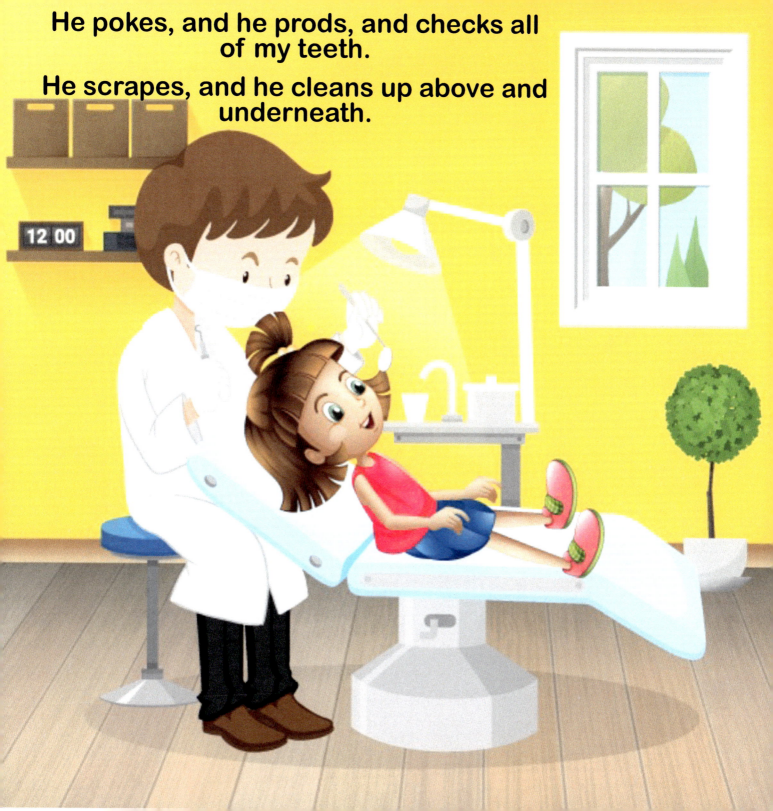

So, you see I've been taking good care of my teeth. My parents remind me and the dentist is pleased.

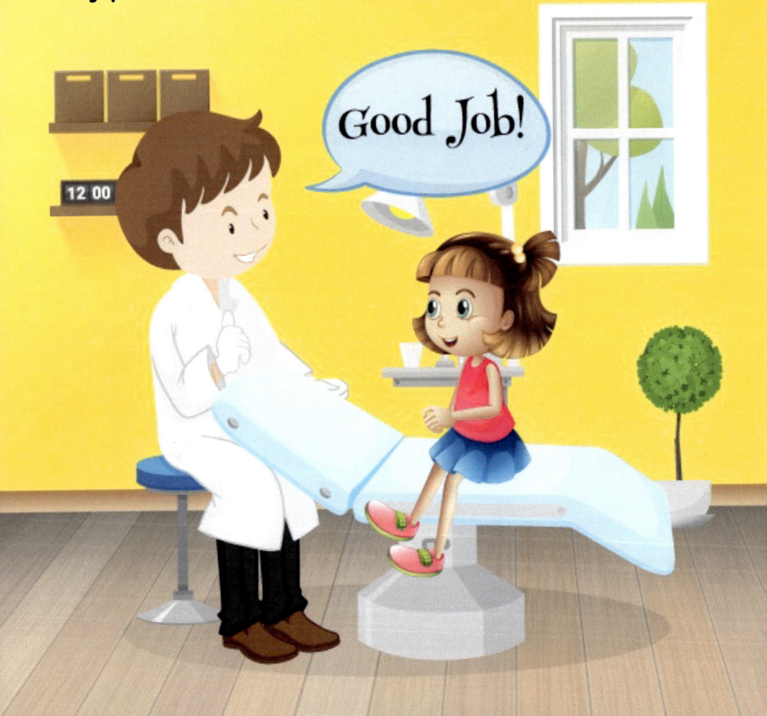

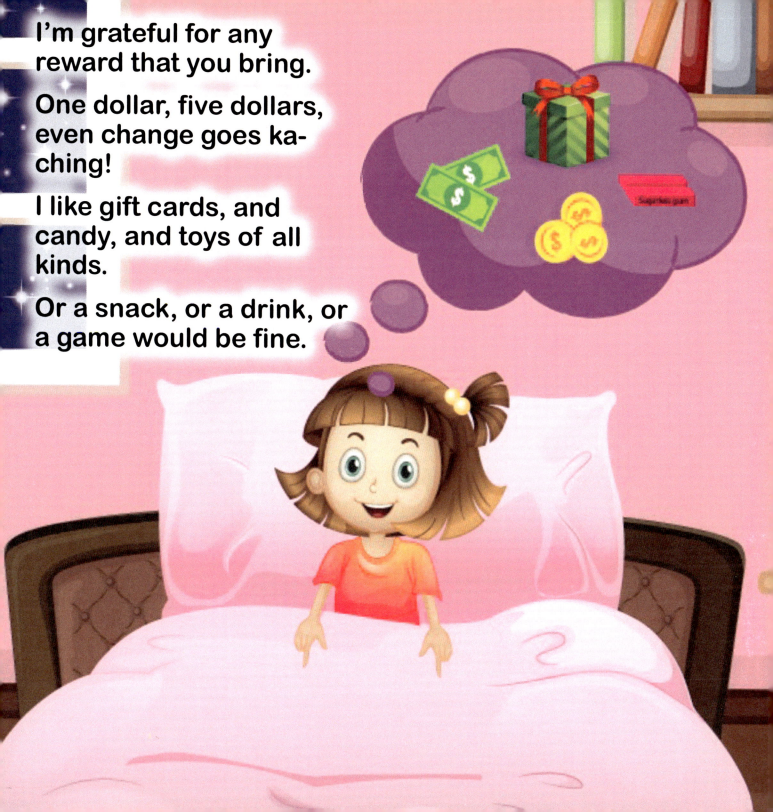

I'm grateful for any reward that you bring.

One dollar, five dollars, even change goes ka-ching!

I like gift cards, and candy, and toys of all kinds.

Or a snack, or a drink, or a game would be fine.

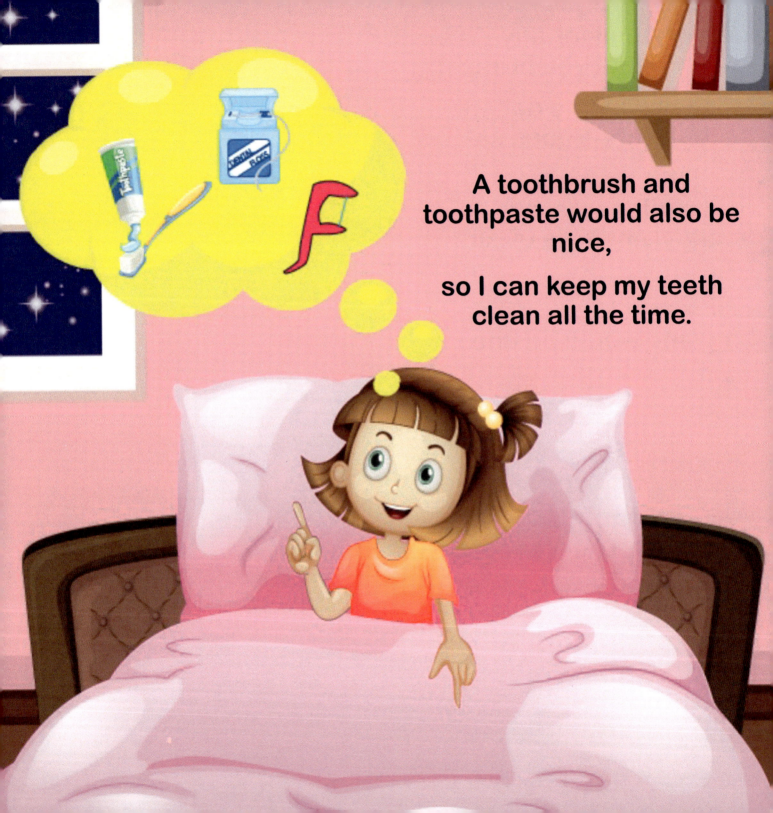

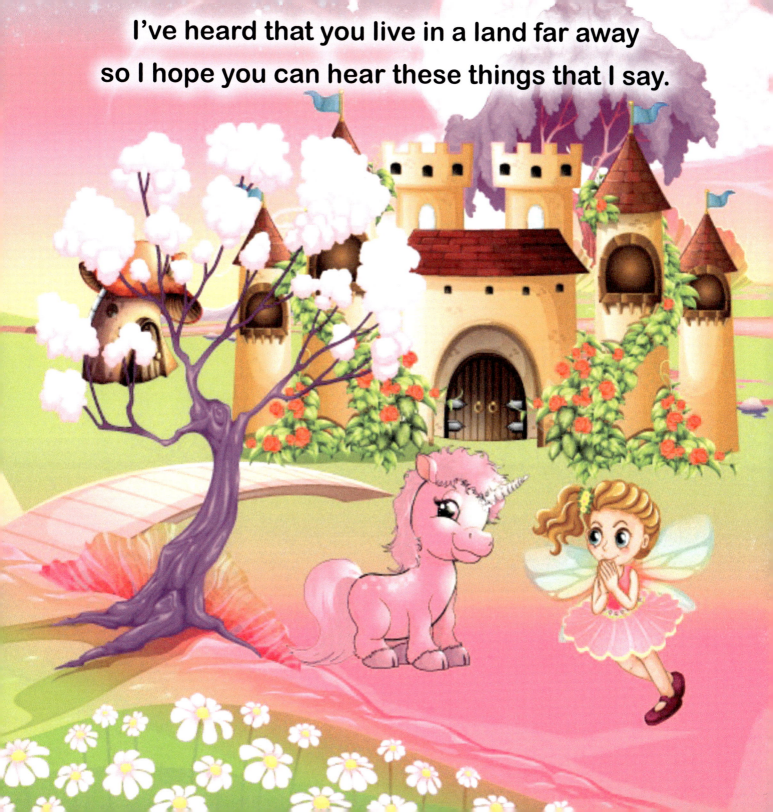

I've heard that you live in a land far away
so I hope you can hear these things that I say.

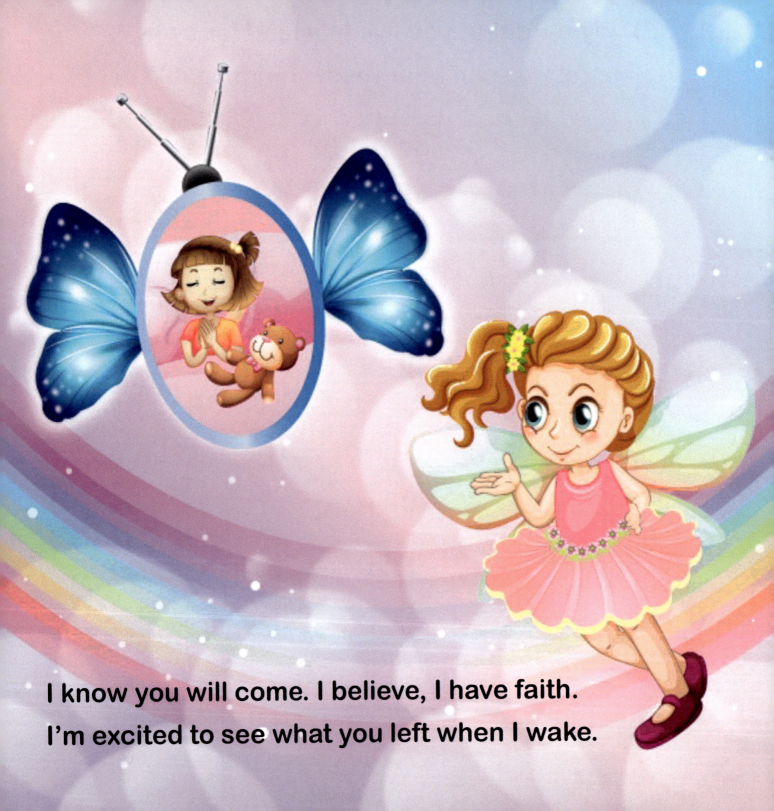

I know you will come. I believe, I have faith.
I'm excited to see what you left when I wake.

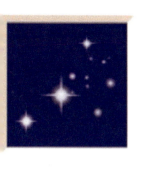

I'm making my wish as I turn off the light.

Oh, tooth fairy, tooth fairy, won't you please come tonight?

The End

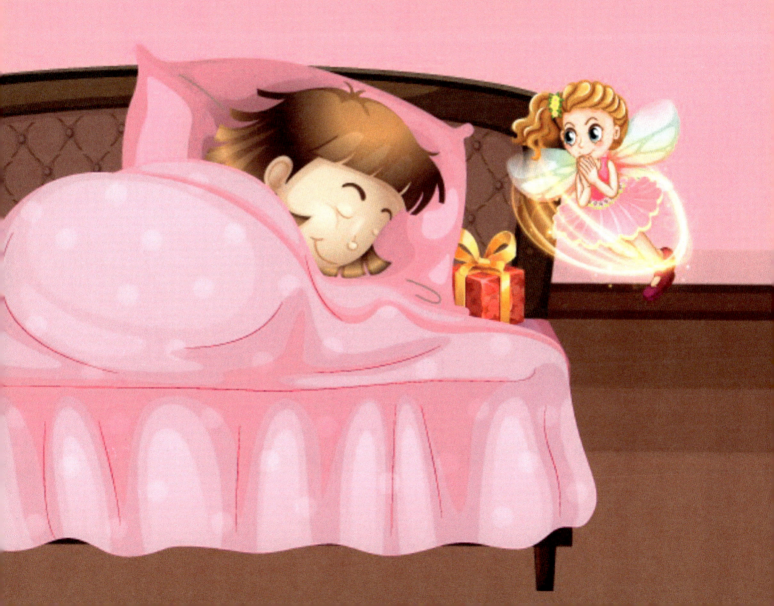

About the Author

André Calbert was born in Northern California and has always been fascinated with the creative arts and the written word. In the mid-2000's he wrote a book about hybrid dog breeds which was published by Barron's Educational Series. André is an avid singer and piano player. He is also a father who has been inspired to write children's books that empower kids in a fun and engaging way. He hopes to share his art with the world, encourage the health and wellness of others, and have a positive impact on humanity.

ToothFairyWishes.com

A Word From The Author

If you enjoyed the book, it would be wonderful if you could take a short minute to leave a kind review on Amazon or whichever website you purchased it on. Your feedback is very much appreciated and so important to help the book be discovered by others who could also benefit. I love to hear stories about your kids and how the book may have encouraged them to brush their teeth, or how much they enjoyed reading it at bedtime. It also encourages me to continue with my upcoming children's books and projects and reminds me of why I do this.

Sincerely,

Andre Calbert

ToothFairyWishes.com

Made in the USA
Monee, IL
06 February 2023

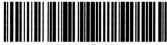